Bridging the Divide

Bridging the Divide

Carina Schroedel

CONTENTS

Epilepsy and Mental Health: Bridging Clinical Gaps

Abstract

Epilepsy, a complex neurological condition characterized by recurrent seizures, intersects profoundly with mental health. Research indicates that individuals with epilepsy are significantly more likely to experience comorbid psychiatric disorders, including depression, anxiety, PTSD, and psychosis. Despite this, mental health conditions are frequently underdiagnosed or misattributed to seizure activity or medication side effects, leading to treatment delays and worsening outcomes.

This paper examines existing literature on psychiatric comorbidities in epilepsy, highlighting biological, psychosocial, and diagnostic overlaps. It further explores gaps in clinical care, such as limited interdisciplinary communication between neurology and mental health providers, and the stigmatization of psychogenic non-epileptic seizures (PNES). A mixed-methods research study is proposed to investigate the prevalence of undiagnosed mental health disorders among adults with epilepsy, and to assess the impact of these conditions on quality of life and treatment adherence.

The goal of this paper is to expose the critical gaps in current practice and advocate for integrative, trauma-informed approaches. Clinical recommendations include the implementation of routine mental health screenings in neurology settings, the development of collaborative care models, and greater education for mental health clinicians on seizure-related disorders. In bridging these disciplines, we can improve outcomes for individuals living with epilepsy and support holistic, person-centered healing.

Literature Review

The intersection of epilepsy and mental health disorders has been increasingly recognized as a critical component of holistic neurological care. Decades of research suggest a significantly elevated prevalence of psychiatric comorbidities among individuals with epilepsy compared to the general population. These comorbidities often go underdiagnosed and undertreated, contributing to increased morbidity, reduced treatment adherence, and poor psychosocial outcomes (Kanner, 2016; Brigo et al., 2020). Despite growing evidence of this bidirectional relationship, clinical integration between neurology and mental health disciplines remains limited, pointing to the need for a comprehensive and interdisciplinary approach to epilepsy care.

Prevalence of Psychiatric Comorbidities in Epilepsy

Depression is the most frequently reported psychiatric condition among individuals with epilepsy. The lifetime prevalence of major depressive disorder in this population is estimated at 30–50%, significantly higher than the general population's rate of approximately 17% (Kanner, 2016; Gandy et al., 2022). Anxiety disorders are similarly prevalent, with studies reporting comorbidity rates ranging from 20% to 40% (Tellez-Zenteno et al., 2007). PTSD and psychosis also appear in elevated rates, particularly among those with temporal or frontal lobe epilepsy (Trimble & Schmitz, 2011).

The impact of these comorbidities is substantial. Depression and anxiety have been found to correlate with increased seizure frequency, diminished medication adherence, and lower health-related quality of life (Boylan et al., 2004). Notably, psychiatric symptoms in individuals with epilepsy are often chronic and cyclical, with evidence suggesting that mental health concerns may precede the onset of seizures in some cases, while in others they emerge as a direct or indirect consequence of epilepsy (Gilliam & Santos, 2006).

Shared Neurobiological Mechanisms

Emerging evidence points to several shared neurobiological underpinnings between epilepsy and psychiatric disorders. These include dysfunctions in the limbic system, particularly the amygdala and hippocampus, which play key roles in emotion regulation and memory consolidation (Devinsky et al., 2019). Neurotransmitter imbalances—such as alterations in GABAergic, serotonergic, and dopaminergic pathways—are implicated in both seizure generation and mood disorders (Rogawski & Löscher, 2004).

Temporal lobe epilepsy (TLE) is of particular interest due to its strong association with affective and psychotic symptoms. Patients with TLE exhibit a higher incidence of depression and interictal dysphoria, and may also experience postictal psychosis—a transient, seizure-related psychotic state characterized by hallucinations, paranoia, and confusion (Trimble & Schmitz, 2011). These symptoms are often misunderstood or minimized in clinical settings.

The Role of Trauma and Psychosocial Stress

In addition to neurological factors, psychosocial dimensions significantly contribute to the psychiatric burden in epilepsy. Individuals with epilepsy often experience chronic stress, social exclusion, and stigma, all of which are associated with negative mental health outcomes (Jacoby et al., 2005). Stigma in particular remains a pervasive and harmful force. It has been linked to decreased help-seeking behavior, medication nonadherence, and internalized shame—especially among adolescents and young adults (Austin et al., 2002).

Trauma histories are also underreported yet highly relevant in this population. For individuals with PNES—a condition involving seizure-like episodes without epileptic activity, often associated with unresolved trauma—invalidating experiences within healthcare settings can retraumatize patients and delay effective treatment (Baslet et al., 2016). Despite these connections, trauma screening is not routinely implemented in epilepsy care.

Diagnostic Challenges and Fragmented Care

One of the most pressing issues in the field is the under-recognition and misattribution of psychiatric symptoms. Mood and anxiety symptoms may be overlooked entirely or attributed to side effects of antiepileptic drugs (AEDs), while more severe presentations (e.g., hallucinations, mood swings) may be confused with ictal or postictal phenomena (Goldstein & Mellers, 2006). This diagnostic ambiguity not only delays psychiatric intervention but may result in inappropriate treatment plans, including unnecessary AED adjustments.

Psychogenic non-epileptic seizures (PNES) represent a unique diagnostic and therapeutic challenge. Although PNES accounts for up to 20% of cases in epilepsy clinics, it remains poorly understood by many clinicians, leading to stigmatization and discontinuity of care (LaFrance et al., 2013). Individuals with PNES are frequently dismissed as "difficult" or "noncompliant," despite the clear links between PNES, unresolved trauma, and dissociation.

Furthermore, patients often find themselves navigating disconnected systems of care. Neurologists may feel unprepared to address mental health needs, while behavioral health providers may lack adequate training in seizure-related phenomena. This lack of integration contributes to a care gap where neither provider feels fully responsible for the patient's mental well-being.

Underutilization of Mental Health Services

Despite the clear prevalence and impact of psychiatric comorbidities, mental health services remain vastly underutilized among individuals with epilepsy. A multinational study by Brigo et al. (2020) found that fewer than one in four epilepsy patients with co-occurring psychiatric conditions receive formal psychological support or therapy. Barriers to care include limited access to behavioral health clinicians within neurology clinics, lack of reimbursement for collaborative care, and ongoing stigma surrounding mental health within medical settings.

Moreover, there is a critical lack of standardized mental health screening in epilepsy clinics. Evidence-based tools such as the PHQ-9 and GAD-7 are infrequently administered, and few epilepsy centers include licensed mental health professionals on their treatment teams (Kwon & Park, 2014). This gap persists despite evidence showing that early detection and treatment of mental health symptoms improve both seizure control and patient satisfaction (Gilliam & Santos, 2006).

Summary

The existing literature paints a compelling picture of the intersection between epilepsy and mental health. The evidence confirms a high prevalence of psychiatric comorbidities, highlights shared neurobiological mechanisms, and underscores the profound impact of trauma, stigma, and fragmented care. Yet despite these insights, meaningful integration between mental health and neurology remains limited in practice. The absence of routine screening, interdisciplinary collaboration, and trauma-informed models of care leaves many patients vulnerable to misdiagnosis, poor treatment outcomes, and persistent emotional distress.

These gaps in clinical practice require urgent attention from both research and policy communities.

Gaps in Diagnosis and Treatment

Clinical Barriers and Systemic Failures in Epilepsy and Mental Health Care

Despite the well-documented association between epilepsy and psychiatric comorbidities, significant gaps persist in both diagnosis and treatment within standard neurological care. These deficits are not solely attributable to a lack of awareness but stem from systemic fragmentation, inadequate training, stigmatization, and a pervasive lack of interdisciplinary collaboration. As a result, many individuals with epilepsy remain undiagnosed or misdiagnosed regarding mental health conditions, often enduring years of unnecessary suffering.

1. Diagnostic Oversights and Attribution Errors

One of the most common clinical oversights involves the misattribution of psychiatric symptoms to epilepsy itself or its pharmacological treatment. Mood instability, irritability, fatigue, and cognitive slowing—hallmarks of both affective disorders and side effects of antiepileptic drugs (AEDs)—are frequently minimized or dismissed by providers (Goldstein & Mellers, 2006). This conflation leads to a pattern in which psychiatric symptoms are either normalized within the context of epilepsy or pathologized as purely neurological, leaving underlying mental health conditions untreated.

Moreover, psychogenic non-epileptic seizures (PNES) continue to pose significant diagnostic challenges. Though PNES is increasingly recognized as a trauma-linked, dissociative phenomenon rather than a "behavioral issue," many patients still experience dismissal from care after diagnosis. A 2020 review found that a majority of individuals diagnosed with PNES are referred out of neurology settings with limited or no follow-up care, despite high rates of PTSD, depression, and suicidal ideation within this group (LaFrance et al., 2013; Baslet et al., 2016). This disconnect reveals not only a misunderstanding of PNES as a clinical entity but also a broader failure to adopt trauma-informed approaches within neurology.

2. Absence of Routine Mental Health Screening in Neurology

Despite ample evidence supporting the use of standardized tools such as the PHQ-9 for depression, GAD-7 for anxiety, and PCL-5 for trauma-related symptoms, these instruments are rarely incorporated into epilepsy care. A review by Kwon and Park (2014) found that fewer than 15% of epilepsy clinics conduct any form of regular mental health assessment. This omission is not due to a lack of screening tools, but rather a lack of training, time, and perceived role responsibility among neurologists.

From a systems perspective, this reflects a broader issue of role siloing. In the absence of integrated behavioral health services, neurologists may feel ethically constrained or clinically unprepared to address psychiatric concerns. Simultaneously, mental health professionals may be unfamiliar with seizure physiology, AED pharmacology, or the unique psychosocial challenges faced by individuals with epilepsy—creating a mutual blind spot in care.

3. Stigma and Provider Bias

Stigma continues to influence provider behavior, often unconsciously. Studies show that both epilepsy and psychiatric illness carry high levels of implicit bias among healthcare professionals, affecting diagnostic accuracy and patient-provider communication (Austin et al., 2002; Jacoby et al., 2005). This is particularly salient in cases of PNES, where clinicians may perceive patients as malingering, noncompliant, or "difficult," thereby diminishing the quality and continuity of care.

Clinicians who lack training in trauma-informed practice may inadvertently retraumatize patients by invalidating their symptoms or by referring them to services without adequate psychoeducation or support. Such experiences erode trust and reduce treatment engagement. In many cases, patients who receive dual stigmatizing labels—such as "epileptic" and "psychiatric"—report poorer experiences and higher dropout rates from both neurology and mental health services (Baslet et al., 2016).

4. Structural Fragmentation Between Disciplines

The division between mental health and neurology is deeply embedded in both clinical culture and healthcare infrastructure. Few epilepsy centers employ embedded behavioral health specialists or social workers, and even fewer participate in collaborative case management with external psychiatric providers. When mental health referrals are made, they often lack continuity, communication, or shared documentation—resulting in a disjointed and inefficient system of care (Brigo et al., 2020).

Furthermore, reimbursement models and institutional silos reinforce this fragmentation. Behavioral health services may not be covered under neurology visits, and vice versa, complicating billing and discouraging collaboration. These administrative barriers compound existing time constraints and limit clinicians' ability to address patients holistically.

5. Lack of Trauma-Informed Education and Training

Despite the high prevalence of trauma among individuals with epilepsy, trauma screening and trauma-informed care are rarely implemented in neurological settings. There is little standardized education on adverse childhood experiences (ACEs), PTSD, or dissociative symptoms in most neurology residencies or continuing education programs. Likewise, behavioral health clinicians often lack training in seizure identification, psychotropic-AED interactions, or seizure first aid—limiting their clinical confidence when working with this population.

Without shared language and cross-disciplinary education, both neurologists and mental health professionals may feel isolated in their ability to treat patients with co-occurring needs. This results in care that is fragmented, reactive, and insufficiently responsive to the full range of patient experiences.

Summary

The current clinical landscape reveals numerous barriers to effective mental health care for individuals with epilepsy, ranging from diagnostic ambiguity and stigmatizing attitudes to structural fragmentation and educational gaps. While the literature increasingly supports integrated, trauma-informed, and interdisciplinary care models, real-world implementation remains limited. These gaps represent not only missed opportunities for improved health outcomes but also ethical concerns regarding equity, dignity, and the right to comprehensive care. Bridging these gaps requires systemic change and clinician-level commitment to collaborative, informed, and human-centered practice.

Proposed Study

Investigating the Relationship Between Mental Health Disorders and Epilepsy: A Mixed-Methods Clinical Study

Purpose and Rationale

Given the consistent evidence of elevated psychiatric comorbidities among individuals with epilepsy—and the persistent fragmentation of care—there remains a critical need for empirical research that explores the lived experience, diagnostic outcomes, and treatment access of this population. The purpose of this proposed study is to examine the prevalence of undiagnosed mental health conditions in adults with epilepsy, assess how these comorbidities affect seizure frequency and treatment adherence, and explore barriers to integrated care from the patient perspective. This study aims to fill a gap in the current literature by combining quantitative data with qualitative insights to offer both statistical and narrative clarity on this issue.

Research Questions

- What is the prevalence of undiagnosed or subclinical depression, anxiety, and PTSD among adults currently receiving treatment for epilepsy?
- How do psychiatric symptoms correlate with seizure frequency, treatment adherence, and perceived quality of life?
- What psychosocial and systemic barriers do individuals with epilepsy face in accessing appropriate mental health care?

- How do patients describe their experiences of stigma, dismissal, or fragmentation in epilepsy and mental health services?

Hypotheses

- **H1:** Adults with epilepsy will show a significantly higher rate of positive screens for depression, anxiety, and PTSD than the general population.

- **H2:** Increased psychiatric symptom severity will be associated with higher reported seizure frequency and lower treatment adherence.

- **H3:** Patients with higher perceived stigma will report lower engagement with both neurology and mental health services.

- **H4:** Qualitative data will reveal consistent themes of dismissal, lack of trauma-informed care, and limited interdisciplinary coordination.

Methodology

Design:

A mixed-methods cross-sectional study incorporating validated mental health screening tools and in-depth qualitative interviews.

Participants:

A total of **100 adults** (ages 18–65) diagnosed with epilepsy and receiving care from outpatient neurology clinics in both urban and rural settings. Participants with confirmed intellectual disabilities or active psychosis will be excluded to ensure reliability of self-report measures.

Recruitment:

Participants will be recruited through neurology clinics, epilepsy foundations, online patient networks, and support groups. Informed consent will be obtained prior to participation.

Instruments:

- **PHQ-9**: Depression screening
- **GAD-7**: Anxiety screening
- **PCL-5**: PTSD screening
- **QOLIE-31**: Quality of Life in Epilepsy inventory
- **Adherence to Medication Scale**
- **Stigma Scale for Chronic Illnesses**

Procedure:

Participants will complete a brief electronic survey (20–30 minutes) including all instruments listed above. A subset (n = 25) will be invited to participate in a 45-minute semi-structured interview exploring themes of stigma, diagnostic experience, trauma history, provider communication, and mental health access.

Data Analysis:

Quantitative data will be analyzed using descriptive statistics, Pearson correlations, and multiple regression analyses to examine relationships between psychiatric symptoms, seizure frequency, and treatment adherence.

Qualitative interviews will be transcribed and coded using thematic analysis to identify recurring themes, unique narratives, and cross-participant patterns related to clinical care experiences.

Expected Outcomes and Impact

This study is expected to demonstrate a high prevalence of unaddressed mental health symptoms among individuals with epilepsy, strong correlations between psychiatric burden and seizure-related outcomes, and a clear need for integrated care models. By incorporating patient voice through qualitative interviews, the study will also shed light on the emotional and systemic challenges individuals face when navigating disjointed care systems.

Findings will inform future recommendations for routine mental health screening in neurology, development of cross-disciplinary provider training, and implementation of trauma-informed, person-centered care models. Results will be disseminated through publication in clinical journals, conference presentations, and patient education channels to advocate for systemic improvements.

Discussion

Bridging the Gap Between Mental Health and Neurology: Toward Integrated, Trauma-Informed Epilepsy Care

The findings from the literature and the proposed research study underscore a significant yet long-neglected intersection between epilepsy and mental health. Despite decades of data affirming high rates of psychiatric comorbidity in individuals with epilepsy, the systems designed to treat these conditions remain siloed, inconsistent, and poorly equipped to offer coordinated care. This disconnect places an undue burden on patients—many of whom must navigate complex medical systems while simultaneously managing unacknowledged psychological distress.

The implications for clinical practice, systems planning, and policy development are substantial. Meaningful improvement in outcomes for individuals with epilepsy cannot occur without the integration of mental health into standard neurological care.

1. Implementing Routine Mental Health Screening in Epilepsy Care

One of the most accessible and effective first steps toward bridging this gap is the implementation of routine mental health screenings in neurology clinics. Brief, validated tools such as the **PHQ-9**, **GAD-7**, and **PCL-5** can be administered at intake or during follow-up visits with minimal burden to clinicians or patients. These tools provide critical insight into psychiatric symptomatology that often remains unspoken or misattributed to seizure disorders or medication side effects.

However, screening must not occur in isolation. Positive findings must be followed by appropriate referrals, collaborative care planning, and clear communication between neurologists and behavioral health providers. Without this infrastructure, screening risks becoming a performative measure rather than a meaningful clinical intervention.

2. Embedding Behavioral Health Professionals in Neurology Settings

Integrated care models, in which behavioral health professionals are embedded within medical clinics, represent a gold standard for addressing co-occurring conditions. While such models are increasingly common in primary care, they remain rare in neurology. Embedding licensed clinical social workers, psychologists, or trauma-informed therapists into epilepsy centers allows for real-time consultation, continuity of care, and interdisciplinary treatment planning.

This approach also facilitates immediate psychoeducation for patients diagnosed with conditions such as PNES, which are often misunderstood or stigmatized. Mental health professionals in these settings can help normalize emotional responses, provide coping tools, and address trauma histories that may be contributing to seizure-like events—thereby improving patient trust and long-term outcomes.

3. Expanding Clinician Training in Trauma-Informed and Interdisciplinary Practice

Both neurologists and mental health providers must be equipped to recognize and respond to the complex interplay between neurological and psychological symptoms. Training programs should include education on:

- The neurobiology of trauma and its relationship to seizure-like activity
- Pharmacologic considerations (e.g., AEDs and psychotropic interactions)
- Recognizing dissociative states and trauma responses
- Cultural considerations and health disparities in epilepsy treatment
- Communicating diagnoses such as PNES in a non-stigmatizing, supportive manner

Continuing education and cross-disciplinary learning opportunities are essential to reducing misdiagnosis, improving treatment engagement, and building professional collaboration.

4. Centering the Patient Voice and Lived Experience

Research and clinical care often overlook the patient's lived experience. Yet narratives gathered from individuals with epilepsy reveal recurring themes of dismissal, fear, shame, and emotional isolation. These are not abstract concerns—they directly impact whether patients adhere to treatment, attend appointments, or disclose symptoms honestly.

Qualitative research that includes patient voices not only enriches the evidence base but also helps dismantle clinical assumptions. Listening to lived experiences is an essential component of trauma-informed care. Providers must approach patients with curiosity rather than certainty, humility rather than authority.

5. Advocating for Policy and Reimbursement Reform

The structural separation between mental health and neurology is reflected in insurance models, reimbursement policies, and service funding. Mental health services are often not reimbursable in specialty medical clinics, creating financial disincentives for integration. Similarly, brief therapeutic interventions delivered by social workers or psychologists within neurology clinics may not be billable at all.

Advocating for revised reimbursement structures, bundled care models, and grant funding for integrated clinics is essential for sustainable change. These reforms will require partnerships among clinicians, researchers, patient advocacy organizations, and policy-makers.

Summary

Addressing the psychiatric comorbidities of epilepsy is not a matter of enhancement—it is a matter of necessity. The fragmented care landscape that currently defines this intersection is inadequate for meeting the complex, layered needs of individuals living with epilepsy. By implementing trauma-informed screening, embedding mental health clinicians, prioritizing interdisciplinary education, and elevating patient voice, the field can begin to close the gap between neurology and behavioral health.

Ultimately, integrated care is not just a best practice; it is an ethical imperative. For clinicians, researchers, and systems leaders alike, the time to act is now.

Conclusion

Toward Ethical and Integrated Care in Epilepsy and Mental Health

The comorbidity of psychiatric disorders among individuals with epilepsy is not an incidental concern—it is a core determinant of patient outcomes, treatment adherence, and long-term quality of life. Despite decades of empirical evidence, these intersections remain poorly addressed in both neurology and mental health systems, leaving patients caught in the space between disciplines. Clinical oversight, diagnostic ambiguity, and stigma continue to compromise care, particularly for vulnerable groups such as those with psychogenic non-epileptic seizures (PNES) or a history of trauma.

Bridging this divide requires more than acknowledgment; it demands systemic and cultural change. Routine mental health screening must become standard practice in epilepsy care. Behavioral health professionals must be included as essential members of neurological teams. Trauma-informed, interdisciplinary education must be integrated into professional training. And above all, the lived experience of those navigating epilepsy and mental health challenges must be valued as central to both research and clinical reform.

As clinicians, researchers, and systems leaders, we are ethically obligated to close these gaps. The path forward lies in integrated, compassionate, and evidence-based care—where no patient is left untreated, misdiagnosed, or dismissed for symptoms that fall between specialties. This is not a future goal. It is an urgent necessity.

Carina Schroedel, CSW, LCADCA is a clinical social worker, addiction counselor, and holistic healing practitioner with over a decade of experience supporting individuals navigating trauma, chronic illness, and emotional recovery. As both a therapist and an individual living with epilepsy, Carina brings a rare and deeply personal insight into the intersection of mental health and neurological care.

She is the founder of *Ember & Ease*, a therapeutic practice devoted to integrative healing—blending evidence-based clinical methods with somatic practices, yoga therapy, and trauma-informed support. Carina's professional work centers on bridging gaps between systems, restoring dignity to underserved populations, and advocating for compassionate, collaborative approaches in behavioral health.

In addition to her clinical roles, she is the author of several published workbooks and mental health resources, and a passionate voice in the epilepsy and recovery communities. *Epilepsy and Mental Health: Bridging Clinical Gaps* reflects both her academic rigor and her lived experience—and stands as a call to action for a more integrated and human-centered model of care.

References

Austin, J. K., Shafer, P. O., & Deering, J. B. (2002). Epilepsy familiarity, knowledge, and perceptions of stigma: Report from a survey of adolescents in the general population. Epilepsy & Behavior, 3(4), 368–375. https://doi.org/10.1016/S1525-5050(02)00004-X

Baslet, G., Dworetzky, B. A., Perez, D. L., & LaFrance, W. C., Jr. (2016). Psychogenic non-epileptic seizures: An updated primer. Psychosomatics, 57(1), 1–17. https://doi.org/10.1016/j.psym.2015.10.002

Boylan, L. S., Flint, L. A., Labovitz, D. L., Jackson, S. C., Starner, K., Devinsky, O. (2004). Depression but not seizure frequency predicts quality of life in treatment-resistant epilepsy. Neurology, 62(2), 258–261. https://doi.org/10.1212/WNL.62.2.258

Brigo, F., Igwe, S. C., Ausserer, H., Nardone, R., Tezzon, F., & Trinka, E. (2020). Why do patients with epilepsy not receive adequate psychiatric treatment? European Journal of Neurology, 27(10), 2008–2016. https://doi.org/10.1111/ene.14327

Devinsky, O., Sacks, O., & Devinsky, J. (2019). Epilepsy and behavior: A neurobiological perspective. Epilepsy & Behavior, 96, 329–336. https://doi.org/10.1016/j.yebeh.2019.04.045

Gandy, M., Sharpe, L., & Simpson, T. (2022). Depression and anxiety in epilepsy: A bidirectional relationship. Clinical Psychology Review, 92, 102108. https://doi.org/10.1016/j.cpr.2022.102108

Gilliam, F. G., & Santos, J. (2006). Diagnosing depression in patients with epilepsy. Epilepsy & Behavior, 8(S1), S1–S7. https://doi.org/10.1016/j.yebeh.2005.10.015

Goldstein, L. H., & Mellers, J. D. C. (2006). Ictal and non-ictal psychiatric disorders in epilepsy: A review. Epilepsy Research, 75(2–3), 113–127. https://doi.org/10.1016/j.eplepsyres.2007.04.013

Jacoby, A., Snape, D., & Baker, G. A. (2005). Epilepsy and social identity: The stigma of a chronic neurological disorder. The Lancet Neurology, 4(3), 171–178. https://doi.org/10.1016/S1474-4422(05)70086-X

Kanner, A. M. (2016). Most antidepressant drugs are safe for patients with epilepsy at therapeutic doses: A review of the evidence. Epilepsy & Behavior, 61, 282–286. https://doi.org/10.1016/j.yebeh.2016.03.006

Kwon, O. Y., & Park, S. P. (2014). Depression and anxiety in people with epilepsy. Journal of Clinical Neurology, 10(3), 175–188. https://doi.org/10.3988/jcn.2014.10.3.175

LaFrance, W. C., Baker, G. A., Duncan, R., Goldstein, L. H., Reuber, M. (2013). Minimum requirements for the diagnosis of psychogenic nonepileptic seizures: A staged approach. Epilepsia, 54(11), 2005–2018. https://doi.org/10.1111/epi.12356

Rogawski, M. A., & Löscher, W. (2004). The neurobiology of antiepileptic drugs. Nature Reviews Neuroscience, 5(7), 553–564. https://doi.org/10.1038/nrn1430

Schmitz, B. (2005). Psychiatric comorbidity and epilepsy. Dialogues in Clinical Neuroscience, 7(1), 47–52. https://doi.org/10.31887/DCNS.2005.7.1/bschmitz

Tellez-Zenteno, J. F., Patten, S. B., Jette, N., Williams, J., & Wiebe, S. (2007). Psychiatric comorbidity in epilepsy: A population-based analysis. Epilepsia, 48(12), 2336–2344. https://doi.org/10.1111/j.1528-1167.2007.01222.x

Thapar, A., Kerr, M., & Harold, G. (2009). Depression in youth with epilepsy: A review. Archives of Disease in Childhood, 94(12), 931–933. https://doi.org/10.1136/adc.2007.134122

Trimble, M. R., & Schmitz, B. (2011). The neuropsychiatry of epilepsy (2nd ed.). Cambridge University Press. https://doi.org/10.1017/CBO9780511973646

World Health Organization. (2022). Epilepsy: Key facts. https://www.who.int/news-room/fact-sheets/detail/epilepsy

www.ingramcontent.com/pod-product-compliance
Lightning Source LLC
LaVergne TN
LVHW031614210926
848480LV00012B/1557
* 9 7 9 8 3 4 9 4 3 4 3 8 9 *